Social Skills Solutions

A Children's Behavioral Health Empowerment Program Model

Created By

Rev. Dr. Geraldine L. Johnson-Carter

"All children have within them the potential to be great kids. It's our job to create a great world where this potential can flourish."

-Stanley Greenspan

The information provided herein is stated to be truthful and consistent, in that any liability, in terms of inattention or otherwise, by any usage or abuse of any policies, processes, or directions contained within is the solitary and utter responsibility of the recipient reader.

Under no circumstances will any legal responsibility or blame be held against the publisher for any reparation, damages, or monetary loss due to the information herein, either directly or indirectly. Respective authors own all copyrights not held by the publisher.

The information herein is offered for informational purposes solely, and is universal as so. The presentation of the information is without contract or any type of guarantee assurance.

The trademarks that are used are without any consent, and the publication of the trademark is without permission or backing by the trademark owner. All trademarks and brands within this book are for clarifying purposes only and are

then owned by the owners themselves, not affiliated with
this document.

Table Of Contents

Introduction   10

Target Population   11

Documentation Of Need   12

Purpose   14

Project Goals   16

Impact Description   17

Outcomes   19

Establishing Participant Engagement   21

Program Evaluation   23

Why Affirmation Cards Are Important   25

THE STORIES

Responsible Behavior   28

Right Vs Wrong   31

Persistence & Mental Strength   34

Importance Of Education   37

Empathy & Cooperation   40

Honesty & Ethics   43

Self-esteem & Confidence   46

Perspective & Perception   49

A Positive Attitude   53

Respect For Eldership & Family Values   56

Perception & Controlling Emotions   60

Values & Gratefulness   63

Friendships & Healthy Behavior   66

Appropriate Behavior & Well-Being   69

Gratefulness & Thankfulness   72

Behavior Management   75

Wisdom & Decision Making   78

Valuing Time & Time Management   82

Non Verbal Communication & Moral Behavior   85

Managing Emotions   88

ASSESSMENTS

Children's Behavioral Health Assessment   92

Adult Behavioral Assessment   95

Adult Behavioral Health Mood Indicator   99

A SOLUTION IS...

S - Supportive

O - Optimistic

L - Loving

U - Understanding

T - Truthful

I - Informative

O - Organized

N - Non-Threatening

PROJECT TITLE:
Social Skills Solutions

Introduction

Social Skills Solutions is a culturally relevant, community based behavioral health program model designed to engage, equip and empower parents, families and organizations (academic and faith based) for working with youth.

This is accomplished by providing highly effective activities that help youth increase their values, morals and ethics so they can build a strong foundation to become successful in life.

The activities within the Social Skills Solutions Program Model promotes self esteem, well being, positive thinking, enhances their ability to deal with stress and recover after traumatic events occur in their personal lives.

Target Population

<u>Population #1</u>. Youth directly in the age range of 5 through 8 years

<u>Population #2</u>. Parents/families that have children ages 5 through 8 involved with community based Organizations/ Agencies

Documentation Of Need

There is a clearly documented need that more and more young children are lacking social skills as they enter academic settings. This need is documented by the alarming increase in the number of children who display "acting out" behavior in their academic settings.

Social skills development activities are needed to prepare these youth to effectively interact and communicate with others in the home and in academic settings. Social skills solutions are needed to assist these youth in gaining an awareness of verbal and non verbal communication.

To teach them the skills of basic speech, gestures, facial expressions and body language. There is also the need to assist adults in understanding that the biggest impact they can have on young children is to help them in developing and learning good social skills.

If social skills are taught and reinforced at an early age youth will have the strong foundation they need as adults to succeed in life. Good social skills are needed for positive interaction with other people and they are a critical element in having youth succeed, socially, emotionally, personally and even academically.

Social skills are the skills and behaviors that help youth to join in conversations, work co-operatively with others, develop lasting friendships, effectively self-advocate when needed, and so much more.

Relevant social skills solution activities will help youth to develop a positive attitude, use good manners, work cooperatively with others, follow directions, have good hygiene, be able to take turns, be a good sport, have patience and practice forgiveness with self and others.

Purpose

Social skills solution stories and positive I AM affirmations are designed to help participants to develop their ability to effectively deal with adversity, deal with the day-to-day stressors in life and to develop positive thinking which leads to better life outcomes.

As youth gain confidence in their ability to face life challenges, they will stretch themselves and develop techniques for self-control and for keeping their emotions in check. Social skills solution stories teach:

-Resilience

-Values

-Morals and ethics

-Conflict resolution

-Empathy

-Respect for self and others

-Effectively communication

I AM affirmations are also used to change the way young children feel about themselves. When children start to think differently they will start to feel differently, take different actions and have more positive behavioral experiences and outcomes.

Project Goals

1. To provide a culturally relevant, community based social skills solution model using an oral tradition story telling process (short, rhyming proverbs) along with I AM affirmation cards to engage, equip and empower parents, families and staff of community agencies and organizations to provide needed social and emotional development for youth 5 through 8 years old.

2. To train needed trainers (TNT) such as parents, family members and community members to implement the social skills solution stories and (I AM) affirmation cards behavioral health impact process.

Impact Description

Storytelling using PROVERBS is a fun and non threatening behavioral health impact process, which is powerful when combined with visual, auditory and kinesthetic (learning through hearing, speaking and physical activity).

Proverbs are short, rhyming, unforgettable stories that teach wisdom principles regarding morality without guilt, blame or shame. Proverbs offer good advice about life and how people should live. Proverbs are easily understood, easy to remember and easy to follow.

I AM affirmations are encouraging reminders of self worth such as I AM enough, I AM lovable, I AM someone important. Affirmations are used to help youth shift their perspective from negative to positive self worth and self esteem.

For the program to become effective, youth should be offered 10 weeks of 1½ hours of involvement which will expose them to 2 proverb stories per week as well as (I AM affirmation cards} with affirming words which are reminders of self worth.

The I Am affirmations are also used to push back fears, doubts, anxiety and insecurity. Parents and or an older family member or assigned community program staff member should be recruited to take part in 5 support sessions.

In these sessions they will learn how to implement the proverbs and positive I AM affirmations in the home and community setting. Social skills solution stories and I AM affirmation are specifically designed to help participants develop an optimistic outlook on life and hope for a positive future.

Outcomes

1. Increase participant's positive communication skills

2. Increase participant's ability to effectively deal with adversity

3. Increase participants ability to deal with day to day stressors in life.

4. Increase participant's positive thinking which leads to better outcomes in life.

5. Increase participant's overall coping skills

6. Increase participant's self worth and self image.

7. Increase participant's understanding of the importance of obtaining a quality education

8. Decrease participant's behavior which lead to social problems.

9. Increase adult awareness of and ability to effectively support youth in gaining appropriate social skills

Establishing Participant Engagement

There should be a call to Action Community engagement meeting held for agencies and organizations who have been identified as serving youth in the age range of the targeted population of 5 through 8 years old. Two groups of 10 youth in each group should be implemented at the same time for 10 weeks.

1. Youth ages 5 and 6 in group and youth ages 7 and 8 in group

2. Parent's of participating youth or a family member, professional and non-professional educators, social service and community based organizations staff and community leaders.

Others from religious groups will have the opportunity to take part in and learn how to utilize the social skills solution model using proverbs and positive I AM affirmations.

There should be 5 training sessions offered over the 10 week period for adults. An informational video should be shared with those interested in taking part in the social skills solution behavioral project model.

It highlights the visual, auditory, and kinesthetic storytelling process that has been time tested and proven to be an effective behavioral health model which will help youth practice and learn new behaviors, learn to trust others and grow to their fullest potential.

Program Evaluation

A pre–post program evidence based assessment (Appendix) should be administered before and after participation in the social skills solution behavioral health program model. The pre-post training measurement tool is designed to examine changes in both values, morals, ethics and knowledge.

There is a 30 question pre–post assessment for children and a 20 question pre-post assessment specific to adults who will receive training and empowerment tools. These self reporting assessments will measure the impact of the Social Skills Solutions program of support.

The self assessments are designed for participant's to self reflect, and be honest and open. The self assessments allow all participants to report on their feelings and emotions without the fear of being judged.

Participants will report on their growth and development or lack there of. Their responses will be valued and respected and noted for effective future programmatic changes and development.

Why Affirmation Cards Are Important

The purpose of an Affirmation card is not to change anything outside of yourself, but to change the way you feel about a specific area of your life. When you feel differently about something you start to think and believe differently about it.

When you think and feel differently, you will choose to take different actions, and as a result positive experiences will manifest into your life. The true power of an affirmation is that it helps you form better beliefs which influence increased positive actions.

The practice of affirmations allows us to begin replacing negative thoughts with more positive ideas and concepts. Even ten minutes a day of repeating effective affirmations can help you challenge and overcome self sabotaging and negative thoughts.

All you need to make affirmations work for you is faith and perseverance. Believe that these words have the power to change your life and they will. Small miracles will start happening in your life as your new positive attitudes start to attract positive experiences.

THE STORIES

Responsible Behavior

STORY: Every Tub Must Sit On It's Own Bottom

One day my Daddy took me on a long walk. He said, "My son, you and I need to talk."

You are a big boy now, and there's something you should know. Especially if you want to succeed as you grow.

As you travel through life you will make mistakes, stumble and fall. Yet you will learn and gain new strength through it all.

"Never deny when you are wrong and say, it's not me," just be a man and accept responsibility."
My Daddy had a lot to say on that day. But one rule he wanted me to learn and obey.

He told me no one always behaves as they should, but he wanted me to try my very best to be good.

He said, "Remember this fact that we all have in common: Every tub must learn to sit on its own bottom."

Step #1: Have someone tell the story back in their own words

Step #2: Explain to the youth that for humans the story means that we must learn to stand on our own two feet and learn how to take care of ourselves and our things. It is important to become self sufficient.

Step #3: Read and ask the questions

Step #4: Have the youth pick an I AM affirmation card and look in the magic mirror to repeat the affirmation. *Group Leader assist children who cannot read or have difficulty reading

The Questions

1. What did the father tell the little boy?

2. What were some of the things that the father told the little boy about traveling through life?

3. Why do you think it is important to learn from your mistakes?

4. What did the boy's father tell him about how people behave?

5. Why is it important to accept responsibility for your behavior?

6. What are some things that you do that show you are responsible?

7. Why is it important to not let failure get you down?

Right Vs Wrong

STORY: Pretty Is As Pretty Does

Pretty is as pretty does, My mother always said, these are things she told me as she tucked me into bed.

Never lie, cheat or steal, and do not follow those that will. Keep your things in their proper place, do this with a happy face.

It does not matter if you're at school or play, say please and thank you, excuse me and you are welcome. Use good manners every day.

Step #1: Have someone retell the story in their own words

Step#2: Share with the youth that "pretty is as pretty does" means that having good behavior is more important than having good looks, whether you are a girl or a boy. If you are a kind, and loving person, you are beautiful. However, even if you are good looking but are not nice to others, then you are not truly a beautiful person.

Step #3: Read and ask the questions

Step #4: Have the youth pick an I AM affirmation card and look in the mirror while repeating the affirmation. *Group Leader assist children who cannot read or have difficulty reading

The Questions

1. What did the mother tell the little girl?

2. What were some of the things the mother told the little girl never to do?

3. Why do you think it is important to always tell the truth?

4. Why do you think the mother did not want the little girl to play with those who lie, cheat and steal?

5. Why do you think it is important to keep your things in their proper place?

6. Why is it important to have a happy face when you are taking care of your own things?

7. What are examples of good manners?

Persistence & Mental Strength

There was an old lady who lived on my street. I would often visit and sit at her feet. She would tell me things that I found to be true.

Some of these things I will now share with you.

Life is not always easy, sometimes you may fail rather than achieve. Don't let that stop you, just continue to believe.

Show no concern for what others may do, but do what you know is best just for you.

When you try as hard as you can. Don't let failure get the upper hand.

If at first you don't succeed. Try again, start over again and next time you will win indeed.

Step#1: Have someone tell the story in their own words.

Step #2: Share with youth that they may not always be successful at what they are trying to do the first time they try. State that success does not always happen immediately but if you keep trying you can usually accomplish your goal.

Step #3: Read and ask the questions

Step #4: Have the youth pick an I AM affirmation card and look in the mirror and repeat it.
*Group Leader assist children who cannot read or have difficulty reading

The Questions

1. Where did the old lady live?

2. Where did the little girl sit when she went to visit the old lady?

3. What are some of the things the old lady told the little girl?

4. What does doing what is best for you mean?

5. What does it mean to start over again?

6. What does it mean to win?

Importance Of Education

STORY: Get Something In Your Head

Get something in your head My grandmother always said. My Granny knew this golden rule because she could not go to school.

She had to struggle day and night just to learn to read and write. When I began to grow and grow, It was then she let me know,

"Go to school," she said, not just to see your friends and play, but to get a good education. Because, the things you learn in school today no one can ever take away.

Step#1: Have someone repeat the story in their own words.

Step #2: Share that get something in your head means to learn, understand, accept and believe learning and getting information is important.

Step #3: Read and ask the questions

Step #4: Have the youth pick an I AM affirmation card and look in the mirror as they read it.
*Group Leader assist children who cannot read or have difficulty reading

The Questions

1. Why did the little girls Grandmother want her to go to school?

2. Do you think the grandmother wanted to go to school when she was young?

3. Do you like being able to go to school?

4. What are some of the things you like about school?

5. What are some of the things you dislike about school?

Empathy & Cooperation

STORY: Be Kind To Everyone

Be kind to everyone, no matter what they've done. Treat everybody fair, It shows them that you care.

When you're angry you must release, then you can help keep peace.

Treat everybody right, no need to fuss and fight.

Be kind to everyone, because you'll find that it's lots of fun.

Step #1: Have someone repeat the story in their own words.

Step #2: Share with youth that be kind to everyone is a way they can show people that they care about them and a way to share their love for others. Showing kindness brings happiness and a sense of well-being.

Step #3: Read and ask the questions

Step #4: Have the youth pick an I AM affirmation card and read the affirmation while looking in the mirror.

*Group Leader assist children who cannot read or have difficulty reading

The Questions

1. What are some things that make you feel happy?

2. What are some things that make you feel sad?

3. What do you do when some of your friends act angry?

4. What do you do when you see someone in your family fighting?

5. What do you do when you see some of your friends acting like they are sad or unhappy?

Honesty & Ethics

STORY: Honesty Is The Best Policy

My daddy warned me and my mamma , too. That telling a lie will get the best of you. I didn't believe them, so I told a great big lie.

I said my baby brother had choked on some pie. They ran to the kitchen to rescue their little son, then I realized the harm my telling a lie had done.

I felt really bad and bowed down my head, it still didn't stop them from sending me to bed.

I've learned to speak the truth in every word I say. To never, ever tell a lie, not even in play. It's right that I be punished, so I'll grow up to be good, and always tell the truth and do the things I should.

No matter what I may face, or how scared I may be, I learned that the truth is now and will always be the best policy!

Step #1: Have someone repeat the story in their own words.

Step #2: Share with youth that honesty is the best policy means that telling the truth is better than lying even when it is hard to do. Share that honesty makes you feel better and when you feel better you act better.

Step #3: Read and ask the questions

Step #4: Have the youth pick an I AM affirmation and read it while looking in the mirror.
*Group Leader assist children who cannot read or have difficulty reading

The Questions

1. Why did the boy tell a lie?

2. What did the boy's mother and father tell him about telling lies?

3. What was the boy's punishment for telling a lie?

4. Have you ever told a lie?

5. Why do you feel it is important to always tell the truth?

Self-esteem & Confidence

STORY: To Your Own Self Be True

It's important to live and welcome each new day. Learn to care about yourself no matter what others may say.

It really does not matter where we live or who we are. Every person in the world can be a "super star".

You do not have to prove yourself to anyone, especially me. But you owe it to yourself to be all that you can be.

Just keep this one very important thing in view. You will never go wrong if to your own self you are always true!

Step #1: Have someone repeat the story in their own words.

Step #2: Share with youth that to your own self be true means one must always do what is right. It means that before you can be honest with anyone, you must be honest

with yourself and even when you are a small child you feel
bad when you are acting bad.

Step #3: Read and ask the questions

Step #4: Have the youth select an I Am affirmation card
and read it while looking in the mirror.
*Group Leader assist children who cannot read or have
difficulty reading

The Questions

1. What did the boy's mother tell him about each new day?

2. What did the boy's mother say about taking care of himself?

3. Do you think you are a superstar?

4. What are some thing's that you can do to make yourself feel good?

5. What are some of the things that you can do to take good care of yourself.

Perspective & Perception

STORY: The Grass Is Greener On The Other Side

I used to stand at our fence with my eyes open wide and stare at the pretty green grass on the other side. When I looked down at the grass on our ground, I found that it looked very ugly and brown.

The pretty green grass made me want to run and play. I just had to get to our neighbor's yard someday. I shared with my sister how good the neighbor's grass looked to me.

"We have the very same grass," she said, "can't you see?" I wanted to play in the yard next door, I really felt the need to explore. One day I climbed over our fence and when I looked down, to my surprise the neighbor's grass now was ugly and brown.

I started playing and chasing a frog, all of a sudden I saw the neighbor's big dog. The dog ran out to me but he was on a rope. The rope stopped him in time and gave me some hope.

Climbing back over the fence was really very hard. But, I finally made it back to my very own yard. Now my yard looked large and clean and to my surprise it looked pretty and green.

To my sister I had to confide, I found out the grass is not always greener on the other side.

Step #1: Have someone repeat the story in their own words.

Step #2: Share with youth that the grass always looks greener on the other side of the fence. This means that what other's may have in their possession, often looks better to us than what we have. It also means that other people like our friends in school, may seem to be doing better than we are but, perhaps they really may not be doing better. It just looks that way to us.

Step #3: Read and ask the questions

Step #4: Have the children pick an I Am affirmation card and read the card looking in the mirror.
*Group Leader assist children who cannot read or have difficulty reading

The Questions

1. Why did the boy want to get into the neighbors yard?

2. What was the surprise in the neighbor's yard?

3. What was the child doing when he discovered the dog?

4. How did the child feel when he saw the dog?

5. Once the child was back in his own yard, how did his yard look?

A Positive Attitude

STORY: Smile And The World Smiles With You

When I was very small and feeling blue, my mother taught me something I will share with you. When you are feeling a little down, remember to smile and not to frown.

If you cry when you are feeling down, no one will want you to hang around.

Mother told me, "Smile when you are in trouble and it will vanish on the double. If you smile when you are in trouble, then it will float away like a bubble."

Step #1: Have someone repeat the story in their own words

Step #2: Share that people like to be around those who are happy and not those who are sad. A smile can work wonders, it is the best way to face a problem because it will chase away fear and hide pain. Even when you meet someone for the first time, if you smile it shows that you are a friendly person.

Step #3: Read and ask the questions

Step #4: Have the youth pick an I AM affirmation card and read it while looking in the mirror.
*Group Leader assist children who cannot read or have difficulty reading

The Questions

1. What should you do when you are feeling sad?

2. What did the girl's mother teach her about a smile?

3. What did the girl's mother tell her to do when she was in trouble?

4. What do you like to do most, smile or frown?

5. Do you like to be around people who always frown?

Respect For Eldership & Family Values

STORY: Respect Your Elders

Respect and value your elders and show them that you care. Don't put it off until tomorrow for they won't always be here.

My grandfather always spent time and talked with me. He wanted me to be the best person I could be.

He taught me some lessons I'll share with you if I may. He said it's important to make good use of each and every day. Grandfather told me "Easy come easy go." He also said, "Remember that you will reap just what you sow."

"Having little in life is better than having nothing at all. Count your blessings each day and always get back up if you fall."

He told me, "There will be problems in this life to face.
But, every problem has a solution if you handle it with
grace."

He said, "Sometimes it might seem easier to do bad things
and say things unkind. But, it's better to do things that are
nice and have peace of mind."

I learned to see life through my grandfather's eyes, To
never give up but keep focused on the prize.

Step #1: Have someone repeat the story in their own
words.

Step #2: Share that respecting your elders means that you
should be polite, say thank you, listen to what they have to
tell you, visit with them and treat them with care.

Step #3: Read and ask the questions

Step #4: Have the youth pick an I AM affirmation card and
look in the mirror while reading it.

*Group Leader assist children who cannot read or have difficulty reading

The Questions

1. Why did the boy say you should tell your elders that you care?

2. What were some of the things the boy's grandfather told him?

3. Do you think that it's easier to do bad things in life than good things?

4. What did the boy learn from his grandfather?

5. Why do you think having little in life is better than having nothing at all?

Perception & Controlling Emotions

STORY: All That Glitters Isn't Gold

"All that glitters isn't gold," my daddy said to me. That is what he told me as he held me on his knee.

One day when out playing, I felt really bold, so I walked down my street searching for gold. Off in the distance I saw something shine.

"It's gold I thought, and soon it will be mine. "As I walked towards it, it moved further away. Soon it was nearly the end of the day.

I looked around and began to shake. It was then I knew I had made a big mistake. I sat right down and began to loudly cry. A nice old man walked by and asked me why.

I told him that, "I had followed the sun because it glittered like gold." All of a sudden it was dark and I was very, very cold.

He smiled at me as he took my hand, "I'll take you back home my fine little man." He pointed out it's not safe for me to roam, and never, ever should I leave home alone.

Now and forever, I really believe what I have been told. I know what my daddy means, all that glitters isn't gold.

Step #1: Have someone repeat the story in their own words.

Step #2: Share that everything that looks good, precious or true does not turn out to be that way. Many times someone or something may not be as valuable as it first appears to be.

Step #3: Read and ask the questions

Step #4: Have the youth pick an I Am affirmation card and read it while looking in the mirror.
*Group Leader assist children who cannot read or have difficulty reading

The Questions

1. What did the boy's father tell him when he held him on his knee.

2. How was the boy feeling when he was playing.

3. What was the boy searching for?

4. What did the boy think was gold?

5. When did the boy find out the sun was not gold?

6. Who helped the boy find his way back home?

7. Do you think it's okay for young children to leave home without asking their parents?

8. Have you ever left home without telling your parents where you were going?

Values & Gratefulness

STORY: Easy Come Easy Go

Easy come, easy go. At least my parents told me so.

One day when walking down the street. I found some money at my feet.

I thought, "Now I can have some fun," so I picked up the money and began to run.

I went right to the candy store to get lots of candy which I adore. "Give me chocolate!" I demanded "Don't try to cheat me or be underhanded."

When I put my hand in my pocket to pay, I found my money had all slipped away. "Oh well, I thought, now I know, Easy come, easy go."

Step #1: Have someone repeat the story in their own words.

Step #2: Share with youth that easy come easy go, means often things that come easy go quickly, especially money when it is easily gotten, it is soon spent or lost.

Step #3: Read and ask the questions.

Step #4: Have the youth pick an I AM affirmation card and read it while looking in the mirror?
*Group Leader assist children who cannot read or have difficulty reading

The Questions

1. What did the boy find in the street?

2. What did the boy want to buy with his money?

3. If you had found the money what would you have wanted to buy with it?

4. How did the boy feel when he found the money?

5. How did the boy feel when he lost the money?

6. How do you think the person who lost the money felt?

Friendships & Healthy Behavior

STORY: Easy Come Easy Go

As I watched the pretty sky, hundreds of birds went flying bye. Blue birds were flying with blue, Red birds flying with red.

I asked my father, was it really true that red birds never fly with blue birds?

As father tucked me into bed, he told me he had always heard it said, "Things like birds and bees, pretty much do just what they please."

An eagle and chicken are both birds, but of them flying together he had never heard.

Both have wings and feathers and things. The eagle can rise up and up to the skies. The chicken can only run around and around on the ground.

So no matter what the weather, birds of a feather always flock together.

Step #1: Have someone repeat the story in their own words.

Step #2: Share with the youth that it has been found, those who share the same interests or like the same things tend to like being together. Have them think about how they like to spend time with friends who may not look like them but, they enjoy the same things they enjoy.

Step #3: Read and ask the questions.

Step #4: Have the youth pick an I AM affirmation card and read it while looking in the mirror.
*Group Leader assist children who cannot read or have difficulty reading

The Questions

1. What would the child watch to study the birds?

2. What were some of the things the child noticed about the birds?

3. What was the father's response about the birds and bees?

4. What did the father tell the child about eagles and chickens?

Appropriate Behavior & Well-Being

STORY: Look Before You Leap

Look before you leap, so you don't end up in a heap. Remember Humpty Dumpty who sat on a wall. He was not careful and had a great fall.

Each and every day plan how to move. Just take your time, you have nothing to prove. Try to do your best in school, follow each and every rule.

Think about the things that you do. Don't let others get the best of you. When you take time to think before you move, you will find your life will really improve.

Step #1: Have someone repeat the story in their own words.

Step #2: Share with youth that look before you leap means be careful and think about what you are going to do before you do it! It is important to be prepared because when you do things before you think through what you are going to do, it can cause a problem.

Step #3: Read and ask the questions.

Step #4: Have youth pick an I Am affirmation card and read it while looking in the mirror.
*Group Leader assist children who cannot read or have difficulty reading

The Questions

1. Why is it important to think about things before you do them?

2. What happened to Humpty Dumpty when he sat on the wall?

3. What does it mean to leap?

4. What are some things to do in school to make sure that you have a good school experience?

5. Should you try to always do your best in school?

6. Why should you not worry about what other people may say about you?

Gratefulness & Thankfulness

STORY: Count Your Blessings

Count your blessings every day, I would always hear my grandmother say.

"Be thankful for the food you eat, for clothes to wear and shoes on your feet."

Be thankful for morning with its light, for rest and shelter of the night.

"Be thankful for health, for love and friend 's, for everything God's goodness sends."

Step #1: Have someone repeat the story in their own words.

Step #2: Share with the youth that counting your blessings is a prayer. To count your blessings means giving thanks for how lucky you are instead of complaining. Share that blessings are gifts given to them by God that cause them to feel happy and not suffer.

Step #3: Read and ask the questions.

Step #4: Have youth pick an I AM affirmation card and read it while looking in the mirror.
*Group Leader assist children who cannot read or have difficulty reading

The Questions

1. Who told the little girl to count her blessings.

2. What were some of the things the grandmother reminded the girl to be thankful for?

3. What are some things you are thankful for?

4. Do you say thanks to your parents for providing you with clothes and food? Do you say thanks to God before eating your food?

5. What are some things you forget to say thank you or things you do not say thank you for?

Behavior Management

STORY: Haste Makes Waste

One day my mother sent me to the store. She just wanted some milk and nothing more. I decided to try and hurry, down the street I did scurry.

When I reached the store I purchased the milk and ran out the door. Back home I ran really fast. Finally, I reached my front door at last.

As I turned the handle to go inside and then with my little sister I did collide. I spilled the milk, needles to say. That really, really did not make my day.

I have always moved so fast that it caused my mother to scold me. I remember now why I have been told – slow down my pace because HASTE MAKES WASTE!

Step #1: Have someone repeat the story in their own words.

Step #2: Share with the youth that doing something too quickly usually causes mistakes that result in time, effort and material being wasted.

Step #3: Read and ask the questions.

Step #4: Have youth pick an I Am affirmation card and look in the mirror while reading.
*Group Leader assist children who cannot read or have difficulty reading

The Questions

1. Where did the boy's mother send him?

2. Do you feel that he was in a rush because he did not want to go to the store?

3. What did the boy go to the store to buy?

4. Why do you think the boy ran into his sister?

5. Do you think the boy felt bad after he wasted the milk?

6. Do you ever do things in a hurry?

7. Do you think that doing things too quickly can lead to mistakes?

Wisdom & Decision Making

I love to laugh, dance, sing and run. Everything I do is lots of fun. I want to play the minute that I am awake, but one day I made a big mistake.

My Mom and Dad were both away, so I decided to stay home from school and play. I went to make myself some toast, because it's what I really like the most.

But, when I reached for the honey jar, my hand moved just a bit too far. The honey came flying through the air, it landed on my head and got all in my hair.
I scrubbed and scrubbed as hard as I could but, no matter how I scrubbed it did no good.

When my parents came home, they saw what I had done. There was no place to hide, no place to run.

I had to tell my mother and my father that I skipped school. They did not punish me as I thought they would.

They told me all that had happened to me was for my very own good.

They told me there is a time to play and a time to go to school. They said they hoped that I had learned this golden rule. Experience is the best teacher!

Step #1: Have someone repeat the story in their own words.

Step #2: Share with the youth that experience is the best teacher. This means that experiences often helps one learn values like right behavior from wrong. An experience is an activity one goes through and hopefully, they learn something from it so if it turns out to be a bad experience, they won't repeat it.

Step #3: Read and ask the questions.

Step #4: Have the youth pick an I AM affirmation card and read it while looking in the mirror.

*Group Leader assist children who cannot read or have difficulty reading

The Questions

1. What did the girl like to do?

2. What was the girl trying to get off the shelf?

3. How did the girl's parents know what she had done?

4. Why do you think the girl's parents did not punish her for skipping school?

5. Do you think the girl's mother and father should have punished her for skipping school?

6. What did the girl's parents tell her about playing and about going to school?

Valuing Time & Time Management

STORY: Time Waits For No One

I love to watch the clock, to hear it go tick tock, I think it's very grand to look at the big and little hand.

The hands on the clock move around its face from sun to sun. Time does not wait for anyone.

Time is always ahead of you, and you will never catch up with time because it is impossible to do.

Use the time you have the best you can every day, because time waits for no one or at least that's what they say.

Step #1: Have someone repeat the story in their own words.

Step #2: Share time waits for no one means that no matter who you are or what you are doing, time continues on, it does not stop. Hopefully, as young people they will learn to spend their time being productive and doing good in school and in their home environment instead of doing nothing and wasting time.

Step #3: Read and ask the questions.

Step #4: Have the youth pick an I AM affirmation card and read it while looking in the mirror.
*Group Leader assist children who cannot read or have difficulty reading

The Questions

1. Why do you think the child likes to watch the clock?

2. What is so special about clocks?

3. Do you think you make good use of your time?

4. What are some ways you make good use of your time.

5. Do your parents set a schedule for you?

6. Do you follow a schedule on your own?

Non Verbal Communication & Moral Behavior

STORY: Eyes Are The Window To The Soul

Your eyes may be big, your eyes may be small, Your eyes are what will tell it all. If you are happy or if you are sad, your eyes will tell if you feel good or bad.

Your eyes have a lot to reveal, Your eyes will show just how you feel.

There is one thing that you should know, The eyes are the window to the soul.

Step #1: Have someone repeat the story in their own words.

Step #2: Share with the youth that the eyes are the window to the soul. This means that by looking into someone's eyes you can tell how they are feeling and if they are happy or sad. Share that by looking into someone eyes you can even see if they are feeling good or feeling bad.

Step #3: Read and ask questions.

Step #4: Have the youth pick an I AM affirmation card and read it while looking in a mirror.
*Group Leader assist children who cannot read or have difficulty reading

The Questions

1. What can you learn from looking in someone's eyes?

2. Do you think you can tell if someone is sick by looking into their eyes

3. Do you think that someone has to have large eyes to look into them and see how they feel?

4. Do you think the color of someone's eyes makes a difference in being able to tell how they feel?

Managing Emotions

STORY: Anger Is The One Letter From Danger

When I get angry I have found , that I am no fun to be around. I use to scream, kick and shout, until I found out what my emotions were all about.

My mother helped me to understand that I must control my anger and take it In hand. She said, "Your emotions are how you think and feel." "You must prevent them from making your life go down hill."

She taught me a little exercise that I will teach to you. This is what she told me that I must do. "When you feel your anger starting to rise, just take a deep breath and close your eyes." "Count slowly 1, 2, 3 and you will feel your anger start to flee and then you will feel really free."

Don't let anger control you, because anger is only one letter away from danger. If you let anger get out of control, you do not know how far it will go. Say "stop to anger, say stop to danger. "

Step #1: Have someone repeat the story in their own words.

Step #2: Share that anger is only one letter away from danger. That means that when one becomes angry their emotions can get out of control. Share with youth that when someone mistreats them or treats them unkind, it's important for them to stay in control of their emotions no matter how others are acting. Share it is important to find ways to control your anger and not let anger control you.

Step #3: Read and ask questions.

Step #4: Have the youth pick an I AM affirmation and read it while looking in the mirror.
*Group Leader assist children who cannot read or have difficulty reading

The Questions

1. When the child in the story got angry how did other feel about him?

2. Who helped him to understand what he must do with his anger?

3. What did his Mother tell him about his emotions?

4. What did his Mother tell him to do?

5. What did his Mother tell him about not letting anger control him?

6. What did his Mother tell him to say to anger and to danger?

ASSESSMENTS

Children's Behavioral Health Assessment

Pre________ Post ________

Name:____

Date:____________________________

Type the test instructions here. For example, instruct the student to read each question carefully, and then write T (True) or F (False).

Circle **True** or **False**:

1. I like going to school

True/False

2. If my friends ask me to skip school I would do it

True/False

3. I would tell a lie to my parents to keep from getting punished

True/False

4. I always take good care of my clothes and my room at home

True/False

5. I will admit it when I do something I know is wrong

True/False

6. I always behave just as I should

True/False

7. If I fail at something at school or home I stop trying to succeed

True/False

8. I always say excuse me, you are welcome, please and thank you

True/False

9. I show concern for my friends when they are sad or unhappy

True/False

10. My life is always easy

True/False

11. I feel good about myself most of the time

True/False

12. I worry about what my friends think about me.

True/False

13. I feel it is important to learn new things at school

True/False

14. I am always kind to everyone even when they are not nice to me

True/False

15. I always tell the truth

True/False

16. I am happy with my life and who I am

True/False

17. I like where my friends live and feel they live better than I do

True/False

18. I smile a lot more than I frown

True/False

19. I do not enjoy being around old people like grand parents

True/False

20. I feel it is better to have a little in life than to have nothing at all

True/False

21. I think that I can solve most of the problems in my life

True/False

22. I would steal something from a store if I thought I would not get caught

True/False

23. All of my friends have to look and think just like me

True/False

24 I am always in a hurry to get things done so I can play and be free

True/False

25. I pray over my food and appreciate the things my parents provide for me

True/False

26. I can tell how people are feeling by looking into their eyes

True/False

27. When I am angry I will do and say anything I feel

True/False

28. I am always late for school and other activities that I do not like

True/False

29. I can talk to my parents when I feel sad or unhappy and they will listen

True/False

30. I have someone to turn to when I feel afraid or sad

True/False

Adult Behavioral Assessment

Pre_________Post_______

This assessment will give group leaders information on parental influence on their children's behavior. Have each participant circle the corresponding answer alongside each question asked.

Name:_____________________

Date:________________

Circle The Correct Response:

My child's values are influenced by their friends only

Always Sometimes Never

I set age appropriate goals with my child

Always Sometimes Never

I have open communication with my child

Always Sometimes Never

I use non verbal communication as well as words with my child

Always Sometimes Never

I place responsibility on my child for age appropriate self care

Always Sometimes Never

I see my child as a leader

Always Sometimes Never

I feel my child has good communication skills

Always Sometimes Never

I reward my child for good attendance and good behavior in school

Always Sometimes Never

I punish my child for lying, cheating or stealing

Always Sometimes Never

I encourage my child to recognize blessings and give thanks

Always Sometimes Never

I encourage my child to use good manners

Always Sometimes Never

I encourage my child to self advocate

Always Sometimes Never

I encourage my child to listen to others as well as express their own view point

Always Sometimes Never

I allow my child to take part in age appropriate decision making activities

Always Sometimes Never

I teach my child to not give up when they fail at something

Always Sometimes Never

I share with my child the importance of getting a good education

Always Sometimes Never

I encourage my child to be kind to everyone

Always Sometimes Never

I discourage my child from trying to keep up with the neighbors and having everything they see other's with

Always Sometimes Never

I stress with my child how important it is to always tell the truth

Always Sometimes Never

My child knows they can always turn to me when they are sad or
unhappy

Always Sometimes Never

Adult Behavioral Health Mood Indicator

Pre______ Post ______

Have each participant circle the corresponding answer alongside each question asked.

Name: **Date:**

Circle The Correct Response:

1. Sad or depressed mood

                                                  Always Sometimes Never

2. Feeling guilty

                                                  Always Sometimes Never

3. Irritable mood

                                                  Always Sometimes Never

4. Less interest or pleasure in social activities

                                                  Always Sometimes Never

5. Withdrawn from or avoid people

                                                  Always Sometimes Never

6. Find it harder than usual to do things

                                                  Always Sometimes Never

7. See myself as worthless

Always Sometimes Never

8. Trouble concentrating

Always Sometimes Never

9. Difficulty making decisions

Always Sometimes Never

10. Suicidal thoughts

Always Sometimes Never

11. Recurrent thoughts of death

Always Sometimes Never

12. Spent time thinking about a suicidal plan

Always Sometimes Never

13. Low self esteem

Always Sometimes Never

14. See the future as hopeless

Always Sometimes Never

15. Self critical thoughts

Always Sometimes Never

16. Tiredness or loss of energy

Always Sometimes Never

17. Significant weight loss or decrease in appetite

Always Sometimes Never

18. Change in sleep pattern, difficulty sleeping more or less than
usual   Always Sometimes Never

19. Wish that I did not have the responsibility of raising my children
                                                  Always Sometimes Never

20. Do not encourage my child to go to school and get a good
education   Always Sometimes Never

THANK YOU FOR READING

If You Received Useful Tools In This Information, Please Give Me A 4-5 Star Rating!

This serves as a reward for an author. It takes hours and months, sometimes years of no pay to put together books for the purpose of sharing information you see as important to the world.

Please just take out a minute of your time and please leave a quick positive review. Thank you tremendously for taking out the time to read this information and knowledge.

If you really took this information seriously and you applied the key principles into your daily life, I KNOW you are seeing results.

So again, I thank you for your interest in learning and any investment in applied knowledge will always be a winning investment.

For More Books By

Rev. Dr. Geraldine L. Johnson-Carter Visit:

amazon.com/author/geraldinejohnsoncarter